Pregnancy Cookbook With Nutritional Information

The Complete Healthy Guide To Optimal Prenatal Nutrition And Real Food For Pregnancy With 30+ Recipes For Your Pregnancy Meal Plan

By Kimberley Garcia

Copyright

Disclaimer

The information provided in "Amazing Pregnancy Cookbook with Nutritional Information" is intended for general informational purposes only. Kimberley Garcia, the author, is a medical practitioner, but the content of this book is not a substitute for professional medical advice, diagnosis, or treatment. It is essential to consult with a qualified healthcare provider for personalized guidance on your pregnancy and nutritional needs.

The author and publisher of this book make no representations or warranties with respect to the accuracy, applicability, or completeness of the contents. They disclaim any liability for any loss or risk, personal or otherwise, which is incurred as a consequence of the use and application, directly or indirectly, of the information presented in this book.

Every effort has been made to ensure that the information in this book is accurate and up to date. However, medical knowledge and guidelines are constantly evolving, and it is advisable to verify any information related to pregnancy and nutrition with reputable sources and healthcare professionals. The author and publisher are not responsible for errors or omissions or for any consequences arising from the use of the information contained in this book.

The recipes and dietary recommendations in this book are suggestions and should be tailored to individual dietary preferences and restrictions. It is important to exercise personal judgment and seek guidance from a healthcare professional or registered dietitian when making dietary choices, especially during pregnancy.

The use of any product or service mentioned in this book is at the reader's own risk, and the author and publisher do not endorse or recommend specific products or services unless explicitly stated. Any product names, trademarks, or brand names mentioned are the property of their respective owners.

By reading this book, you acknowledge and agree to the terms and conditions of this disclaimer.

About The Author

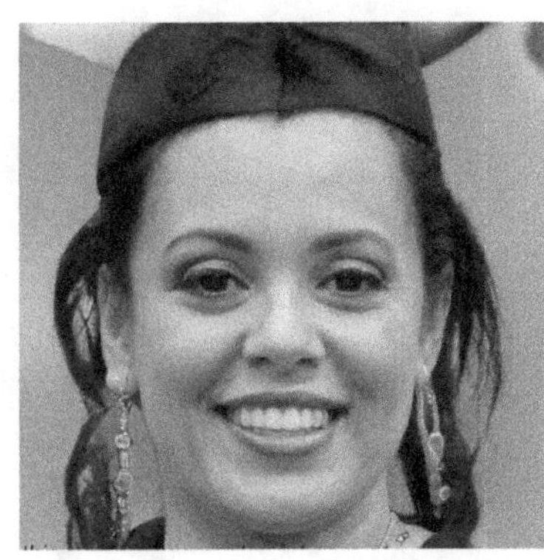

Kimberley Garcia is not only a seasoned medical practitioner but also a passionate advocate for the well-being of expectant mothers and their families. As a dedicated healthcare professional, she has spent years in the medical field, guiding countless individuals on their journeys to better health. Through her knowledge and experience, she has witnessed the profound impact of proper nutrition during pregnancy and understands the vital role it plays in ensuring the health and happiness of mothers and their little ones.

Beyond her professional accolades, Kimberley Garcia is a loving wife, sharing her life's journey with her supportive partner. This personal connection to family life has provided her with a deep understanding of the importance of balanced nutrition and its impact on the well-being of both mothers and their families.

With a passion for education and a desire to make a positive difference in the lives of expectant mothers, Kimberley Garcia embarked on the writing of "Pregnancy Cookbook with Nutritional Information." Her goal is to empower mothers-to-be with knowledge, delicious recipes, and practical guidance, enabling them to navigate the beautiful yet sometimes challenging path of pregnancy with confidence and joy.

Kimberley believes in the profound connection between what we eat and our overall health. Her dedication to bridging the gap between medical knowledge and everyday life shines through in her writing, which is both informative and accessible. She aspires to help you make informed choices about your nutrition, transforming your pregnancy journey into a time of nourishment, vitality, and boundless excitement.

As you delve into the pages of "Pregnancy Cookbook with Nutritional Information," you're guided by Kimberley's expertise, experience, and genuine care. It's her sincere hope that the knowledge and recipes within this book enhance your journey, allowing you to cherish the precious moments of pregnancy and experience the wonder of creating a healthy future for you and your growing family.

Table Of Contents

INTRODUCTION

Pregnancy is a remarkable journey filled with anticipation, joy, and the promise of a new life. It's a time of incredible transformation, not only for your body but for your entire life. As you embark on this path, one thing becomes abundantly clear: the choices you make during these nine months have a profound impact, not only on your own well-being but also on the health and development of your precious, soon-to-arrive baby.

"Pregnancy Cookbook with Nutritional Information" is your trusted guide on this remarkable voyage. This book is a celebration of the power of nutrition, one that can shape the future of your family, starting with the very first moments of life. Our journey together will encompass the knowledge, recipes, and guidance needed to navigate the world of prenatal nutrition.

A Pioneering Adventure in Prenatal Nutrition

Pregnancy nutrition is not just about cravings and food aversions; it's about nourishing your body and your baby in the best possible way. It's about understanding the profound influence your food choices can have on the growth and development of your child.

This book is more than just a collection of recipes; it's a comprehensive resource designed to empower you with the knowledge and tools to make informed choices for a healthy and happy pregnancy. We'll explore the critical role of specific nutrients, the importance of prenatal vitamins, and the advantages of following a pregnancy meal plan tailored to your unique needs.

Your Nutritional Companion

Throughout the chapters of this book, you will embark on a journey of discovery. You'll learn about the vital nutrients required during pregnancy, discover the foods that provide these nutrients, and uncover the secrets to balanced and satisfying meals that support both your well-being and your baby's development.

Whether you're a first-time mom or adding to your family, this book is your companion on the path to a vibrant and nourishing pregnancy. Expectant fathers, partners, and family members are also encouraged to join in, as supporting an expectant mom's nutrition journey is a collective effort.

We believe in the power of knowledge and in the joy that comes from savoring a delicious, nutrient-packed meal. So, let's dive into the world of pregnancy nutrition, one bite at a time. Together, we'll embrace the wonder of this incredible journey, and with the right nourishment, we'll help you embark on the path to a healthy and vibrant future for you and your growing family.

How To Use This Book

Congratulations on choosing "Pregnancy Cookbook with Nutritional Information" as your guide to a healthy and nourishing pregnancy journey. This book is designed to empower you with essential knowledge, practical advice, and a collection of delicious recipes to support your well-being during pregnancy. Here's how to make the most of this resource:

1. **Start with the Introduction**:
Begin by reading the introduction of the book to get an overview of what to expect. The introduction sets the tone and purpose of the book, emphasizing the significance of nutrition during pregnancy.

2. **Progress Through the Chapters**:
The book is divided into chapters, each dedicated to a specific aspect of prenatal nutrition. It's recommended to read through the chapters in order, as they provide a structured approach to understanding and implementing healthy nutrition during pregnancy.

3. **Focus on Knowledge and Nutritional Insights**:
Pay close attention to Chapter 1, where you'll gain a foundational understanding of prenatal nutrition. Here, you'll learn about the importance of specific nutrients, and how they contribute to a healthy pregnancy.

4. **Explore Prenatal Vitamins and Meal Planning**:

Chapters 3 and 4 offer valuable insights into the role of prenatal vitamins and the benefits of a pregnancy meal plan. These chapters provide practical advice and considerations for making informed choices.

5. **Dive into the Recipes**:

Chapter 5 is a treasure trove of 30+ recipes tailored to meet your nutritional needs during pregnancy. Each recipe is carefully crafted to be both delicious and nutritious. You can explore a variety of meals, from breakfast to dinner and even special occasions.

6. **Personalize Your Pregnancy Nutrition**:

While the book provides a wealth of information, remember that every pregnancy is unique. Use the knowledge you gain to adapt the recipes and guidelines to your specific preferences and dietary needs.

7. **Consult with Healthcare Professionals**:

Throughout your pregnancy, it's essential to maintain open communication with your healthcare provider. They can provide personalized advice and address any specific medical concerns you may have.

8. **Enjoy the Journey**:

Pregnancy is a special time in your life, and it's essential to savor every moment. This book is here to support you in making informed and nourishing choices for yourself and your baby. Embrace the journey, celebrate the wonder of life, and nourish your body with love and care.

Remember that "Pregnancy Cookbook with Nutritional Information" is a valuable resource, but it should complement, not replace, the guidance of your healthcare provider. Your healthcare provider is your primary source of personalized medical advice during pregnancy.

KNOWLEDGE OF PRENATAL NUTRITION

Pregnancy is a transforming journey, and it's a time when the nutritional choices you make have a big influence on both your health and the growth of your growing kid. In this chapter, we will discuss the essential components of prenatal nutrition and why it's vital for a healthy pregnancy.

Understanding the Importance of Prenatal Nutrition

Pregnancy is a period of fast growth and development, making it vital for pregnant moms to pay special attention to their nutritional diet. Proper prenatal nutrition offers the building blocks essential for the proper development of your baby's organs, tissues, and overall well-being.

During pregnancy, your body endures a variety of changes, from increased blood volume to hormonal shifts, all of which require extra nutrients to maintain your health and that of your kid. These critical nutrients play a role in avoiding birth abnormalities, maintaining appropriate brain and spinal cord development, and sustaining a healthy birth weight.

Key Nutrients for a Healthy Pregnancy

A balanced and nutrient-rich diet is the cornerstone of prenatal nutrition. The important nutrients you need to focus on throughout pregnancy include:

1. **Folic Acid**: Often referred to as the "superhero" vitamin, folic acid is vital for avoiding neural tube abnormalities in the early stages of embryonic development.

2. **Iron**: Pregnancy increases your blood volume, and iron is vital for carrying oxygen to both you and the baby. Anemia is a prevalent issue, and we'll examine measures to prevent it.

3. **Calcium**: For healthy bones and teeth, calcium is necessary. It also plays a role in muscle and nerve function for both you and your kid.

4. **Omega-3 Fatty Acids**: These healthy fats enhance brain development and eyesight in your child and may lessen the chance of premature delivery.

5. **Protein**: Adequate protein consumption is necessary for the growth and repair of tissues in both your body and your baby's.

6. **Fiber**: Maintaining healthy digestion during pregnancy is vital, and fiber-rich meals aid in this respect.

NUTRITIONAL BUILDING BLOCKS OF A HEALTHY PREGNANCY

Pregnancy is a transforming era in a woman's life, defined by remarkable changes in her body and the quick growth of a new life. These astounding developments are not only the result of nature's magic; they are tightly tied to the critical nutrients that serve as the building blocks of a healthy pregnancy. In this chapter, we will review the main dietary components that underlie a vigorous and successful journey through pregnancy.

Folic Acid: The Foundation of Fetal Development

At the very beginning of this incredible voyage, folic acid takes center stage. Often referred to as vitamin B9, folic acid serves a key function in avoiding neural tube abnormalities during the early stages of embryonic development. This vital vitamin contributes to the creation of the neural tube, which ultimately forms the baby's brain and spinal cord. We will review the recommended daily dose of folic acid and the best dietary sources to ensure you and your baby receive this crucial vitamin.

Iron and Pregnancy: Preventing Anemia

As pregnancy progresses, so does the requirement for iron. Iron is vital for delivering oxygen through the blood, aiding both you and your growing baby. The increase in blood volume during pregnancy means that iron needs grow dramatically, and insufficiency can lead to anemia. We will go into measures to avoid anemia, including dietary sources of iron and implications for iron supplementation.

Calcium for Strong Bones and Teeth

Calcium, a mineral renowned for its role in keeping healthy bones and teeth, is equally crucial during pregnancy. Your baby's developing bones and teeth require a regular supply of calcium, and if your intake is insufficient, your body will sacrifice its own calcium stores to satisfy the requirement. We will investigate ways to satisfy your calcium needs throughout pregnancy, whether you're a dairy aficionado or adopting a dairy-free diet.

Omega-3 Fatty Acids for Brain Development

Omega-3 fatty acids, especially docosahexaenoic acid (DHA), are crucial for the development of your baby's brain and eyesight. These healthy fats have a critical role in promoting the growth of the central nervous system and guaranteeing appropriate brain function. We will examine the necessity of omega-3s throughout pregnancy, sources of DHA, and the function of supplementation if necessary.

Protein for Growth and Repair

Protein is widely praised as the "building block" nutrient, and it plays a key function in pregnancy. Proteins are needed for the growth and repair of tissues, a process that's in high demand as your baby develops. We will review the recommended protein consumption during pregnancy and give a choice of protein sources for both vegetarian and non-vegetarian moms-to-be.

Fiber and Healthy Digestion during Pregnancy

Maintaining strong digestion throughout pregnancy is vital for your comfort and general well-being. Fiber is a food that leads to regular bowel movements and helps reduce typical pregnancy discomforts such as constipation. We'll cover how to add fiber-rich foods into your diet and provide techniques for encouraging good digestion during your pregnancy.

WHAT TO KNOW ABOUT PRENATAL VITAMINS AND SUPPLEMENTS

Pregnancy is a period of heightened dietary needs as your body works relentlessly to nourish both you and your growing baby. While a well-balanced diet is the cornerstone of excellent prenatal nutrition, there are circumstances where dietary consumption alone may not deliver all the critical nutrients your body requires. That's where prenatal vitamins and supplements come into play, providing vital complements to support your health and the growth of your child.

The Role of Prenatal Vitamins

Prenatal vitamins are customized supplements developed to fulfill the particular nutritional needs of pregnant moms. They are not designed to replace a healthy diet but rather to enhance it by supplying important nutrients that may be lacking in your regular meals. Here's what you should know about the importance of prenatal vitamins:

1. **Filling Nutritional Gaps**: Prenatal vitamins are meant to replace nutritional gaps in your diet, especially with relation to minerals like folic acid, iron, calcium, and vitamin D. These are vital for your health and your baby's growth.

2. **Avoiding Birth Abnormalities**: Adequate consumption of folic acid, in particular, has a key role in avoiding neural tube abnormalities in the early stages of pregnancy. Prenatal vitamins guarantee you obtain the appropriate daily quantity.

3. **Supporting Infant's Growth**: The dietary requirements of your developing infant are enormous. Prenatal vitamins are developed to supply the required nutrients to promote embryonic growth and development, from bones to the brain.

Choosing the Right Prenatal Vitamin for You

Not all prenatal vitamins are made equal, and picking the correct one for your requirements is vital. Here are some factors when picking a prenatal vitamin:

1. **Consult Your Healthcare Provider**: Always consult with your healthcare provider before taking any new supplement. They can give information on the specific nutrients you may require and prescribe a suitable prenatal vitamin.

2. **Look for Essential Nutrients**: Check the label of the prenatal vitamin to verify it has critical nutrients such as folic acid, iron, calcium, vitamin D, and omega-3 fatty acids (DHA and EPA).

3. **Consider Special Requirements**: If you have dietary limitations, such as being vegetarian or vegan, or if you have special health issues, such as gestational diabetes, you may require tailored supplements. Your healthcare practitioner can advise on these unique requirements.

4. **Understand Allergen Information**: Pay attention to possible allergies and sensitivities. Some prenatal vitamins may include allergens like as gluten or shellfish, so it's vital to pick a product that corresponds with your dietary restrictions.

Supplementary Nutrients: DHA, Iron, and More

In addition to prenatal vitamins, there may be a requirement for particular supplements during pregnancy. These extra nutrients can include:

1. **Docosahexaenoic Acid (DHA)**: DHA is an omega-3 fatty acid vital for the development of your baby's brain and eyes. It's typically offered as a standalone supplement or incorporated in certain prenatal vitamins.

2. **Iron**: While prenatal vitamins normally contain iron, some women may require extra iron supplements if they are at risk of or are developing iron-deficiency anemia.

3. **Calcium and Vitamin D**: If you don't get enough calcium and vitamin D from your diet or prenatal vitamin, your healthcare practitioner may suggest supplements to maintain bone health.

WHY SHOULD YOU USE A PREGNANCY MEAL PLAN?

Pregnancy brings about a myriad of changes in your life, and one of the most major modifications is in your dietary demands. The decisions you make about what you consume during these nine months have a direct influence not only on your health but also on the growth and well-being of your kid. This is where the notion of a pregnant food plan comes into play—a crucial tool that may convert your prenatal journey into a fulfilling and pleasant one.

Benefits of Following a Pregnancy Meal Plan

1. **Optimal Nutrition**: Pregnancy meal plans are particularly developed to guarantee that you acquire the proper combination of nutrients that are vital for your health and the growth of your baby. With a well-crafted meal plan, you can be certain that you're reaching your nutritional requirements.

2. **Preventing Nutritional Gaps**: Pregnancy is a period when the need for particular nutrients, such as folic acid and iron, increases dramatically. A meal plan helps eliminate nutritional gaps by offering suggestions on which foods to include to fulfill these greater demands.

3. **Balanced Energy Levels**: The hormonal changes that accompany pregnancy might contribute to swings in your energy levels. A pregnant meal plan can help regulate your blood sugar, decreasing energy dips and surges, and ensuring you have continuous energy throughout the day.

4. **Managing Weight Gain**: While weight gain is a natural aspect of pregnancy, a food plan can help you control it more efficiently. By concentrating on nutrient-dense meals and portion management, you may achieve a balance that promotes a healthy weight increase.

5. **Minimizing Discomfort**: Pregnancy can bring along discomforts including heartburn, constipation, and nausea. A well-structured meal plan can give techniques to reduce these

discomforts, such as avoiding trigger foods and integrating products that relieve digestive troubles.

6. **Satisfying Desires**: Pregnancy frequently comes with distinct and sometimes surprising eating desires. A meal plan may meet your cravings within a framework of balanced nutrition, enabling you to enjoy your favorite foods in moderation.

Tailoring Your Meal Plan to Your Unique Needs

It's crucial to recognize that a one-size-fits-all approach to pregnant meal planning may not be the most successful. Every pregnancy is unique, and individual dietary requirements might vary. A tailored meal plan considers your dietary choices, cultural factors, and any medical issues that need particular care.

Planning for Special Dietary Requirements

If you have certain dietary limitations or preferences, such as being vegetarian, vegan, or following a gluten-free diet, a pregnant meal plan may be altered to correspond with your choices while ensuring you still obtain the important nutrients for a successful pregnancy.

Managing Pregnancy Symptoms with Meal Planning

Meal planning also plays a vital part in treating typical pregnancy discomfort. From morning sickness to food aversions, a well-structured meal plan can give solutions and alternatives to help you manage these problems more effectively.

Having a pregnant food plan might help you get through the week. On average, the meals in this diet supply roughly 2,200 calories a day. Read on for single-serving dishes for breakfast, lunch, supper, two snacks (one calcium-rich), and a treat.

30+ RECIPES FOR YOUR PREGNANCY MEAL PLAN

BREAKFAST

Breakfast 1: Classic Apple-Cinnamon Overnight Oats

Remembering to cook these oats before bed may not be simple, but you'll adore waking up to a pre-made meal.

Nutrition Facts

Calories: 448.3

Protein: 19.6g

Carbohydrate: 65.3g

Dietary Fiber: 9.148g

Total Sugars: 24.2g

Total Fat: 13.8g

Saturated Fat: 1.84g

Cholesterol: 4.94mg

Total Omega-3 FA: 1.43g

Calcium: 560.1mg

Iron: 3.147mg

Sodium: 132.1mg

Vitamin D: 0 mg

Folate: 47.7mcg

Folic Acid: 0mcg

Procedure

Pour 1 cup of nonfat milk over 2/3 cup of rolled oats and stir in 1/4 teaspoon of cinnamon.

Cover with plastic wrap and let sit in the fridge overnight.

In the morning, add 2 tablespoons of chopped walnuts and a small, chopped apple.

Breakfast 2: Egg Wrap

Craving some Mexican food? This pregnancy recipe will satisfy your early-morning hunger!

Nutrition Facts

Calories: 453.4

Protein: 26.2g

Carbohydrate: 44g

Dietary Fiber: 6.86g

Total Sugars: 0.941g

Total Fat: 21.2g

Saturated Fat: 5.989g

Cholesterol: 231.5mg

Total Omega-3 FA: 0.164g

Calcium: 353.8mg

Iron: 4.448mg

Sodium: 856.6mg

Vitamin D: 0.438 mcg

Folate: 123.6mcg

Folic Acid: 16.8 mcg

Procedure

Scramble one egg and one egg white in 2 teaspoons of olive oil.

Add 1 cup baby spinach and sauté until just wilted.

Put the egg-spinach mixture on a 10-inch whole wheat tortilla, along with 1/4 cup reduced-fat shredded Mexican blend cheese and 1/4 cup salsa.

Roll up and enjoy!

Breakfast 3: Pear and Cheese Breakfast Sandwich

An English muffin turns this traditional lunchtime sandwich into a fun breakfast option.

Nutrition Facts

Calories: 447.5

Protein: 15.1g

Carbohydrate: 64.5g

Dietary Fiber: 12.6g

Total Sugars: 23.2g

Total Fat: 17.5g

Saturated Fat: 6.914g

Cholesterol: 29.8mg

Total Omega-3 FA: 0.149g

Calcium: 314.7mg

Iron: 2.688mg

Sodium: 397.9mg

Vitamin D: 0.085 mcg

Folate: 88.7mcg

Folic Acid: 0mcg

Procedure

Separate the two sides of a whole wheat English muffin.

Place 1/2 of a large pear, sliced, on one half and top with a 1-ounce slice of cheddar cheese.

Put both halves under the broiler for 2–3 minutes, until the top browns and the cheese is melted.

Sandwich the two halves together. Serve with the remaining half of the pear spread with 2 teaspoons of almond butter.

Breakfast 4: Crunchy Pumpkin Spice Parfait

This pregnancy meal is so tasty that it practically doubles as a dessert.

Nutrition Facts

Calories: 455.4

Protein: 20.7g

Carbohydrate: 68g

Dietary Fiber: 6.357g

Total Sugars: 21.9g

Total Fat: 13.7g

Saturated Fat: 2.825g

Cholesterol: 4.41mg

Total Omega-3 FA: 0.027g

Calcium: 552.2mg

Iron: 3.727mg

Sodium: 199.5mg

Vitamin D: 0mcg

Folate: 71.2mcg

Folic Acid: 0mcg

Procedure

Stir 1/3 cup canned pumpkin puree (not pumpkin pie filling), 1/4 teaspoon pumpkin pie spice, and 2 teaspoons maple syrup into 1 cup of nonfat plain yogurt.

Put half of the pumpkin-yogurt mixture into a mug or glass, top with 2 tablespoons granola, 1 tablespoon raisins, and 2 teaspoons chopped cashews.

Pour on the remaining yogurt mixture and top with another 2 tablespoons granola, 1 tablespoon raisins, and 2 teaspoons chopped cashews.

Breakfast 5: Bacon and Egg Frittata

With this baked dish, you get two breakfast faves—bacon and eggs—in one portable package.

Nutrition Facts

Calories: 184

Protein: 16g

Carbohydrate: 1g

Fiber: 0g

Fat: 11g

Saturated fat: 4g

Sugars: 0g

Calcium: 38mg

Sodium: 456mg

Procedure

Preheat the oven to 350 F. In a medium bowl, whisk together eight eggs with 1/4 teaspoon salt and freshly ground pepper to taste; set aside.

Cook and stir 1/4 pound chopped lower-sodium bacon in a 10-inch non-stick, oven-safe skillet over medium until crisp.

Pour the eggs over the remaining bacon in a skillet. Sprinkle evenly with 1 tablespoon of finely chopped chives.

Transfer the skillet to the oven and bake for 10–12 minutes or until set.

This recipe makes eight servings. Serve warm, cold, or at room temperature. Refrigerate for up to three days. Enjoy this pregnancy recipe with a medium (16-ounce) nonfat decaf latte and an orange.

LUNCH

Lunch 1: Egg-cellent Veggie and Hummus Pita

This pita has veggies, eggs, hummus, and tons of flavor!

Nutrition Facts

Calories: 553.8

Protein: 22.4g

Carbohydrate: 81.1g

Dietary Fiber: 9.963g

Total Sugars: 28.3g

Total Fat: 18.5g

Saturated Fat: 3.116g

Cholesterol: 212mg

Total Omega-3 FA: 0.172g

Calcium: 104.6mg

Iron: 5.154mg

Sodium: 620.7mg

Vitamin D: 0 mg

Folate: 125.4mcg

Folic Acid: 0 mg

Procedure

Fill a 6-inch whole wheat pita with 1/4 cup hummus, one sliced hard-boiled egg plus one hard-boiled egg white, 1/3 cup chopped tomato, 1/2 cup baby spinach, a sprinkle of paprika, and 1 tablespoon toasted pine nuts.

Serve with a cup of grapes.

Lunch 2: Colorful Crab Salad Sandwich

While some seafood is off-limits during pregnancy, you can indulge in your cravings with this safe and tasty crab salad sandwich.

Nutrition Facts

Calories: 564.4

Protein: 33.2g

Carbohydrate: 69.6g

Dietary Fiber: 11.9g

Total Sugars: 9.441g

Total Fat: 20.8g

Saturated Fat: 2.286g

Cholesterol: 110.5mg

Total Omega-3 FA: 1.186g

Calcium: 183.2mg

Iron: 6.462mg

Sodium: 1103mg

Vitamin D: 0 mg

Folate: 87.6mcg

Folic Acid: 0mcg

Procedure

Mix a 6-ounce can of crab meat (drained) with 2 tablespoons light mayonnaise, 1/4 cup shredded carrot, 1/4 cup diced celery, and 1 tablespoon chopped red onion. Spread the mixture onto a slice of whole wheat bread and top with a second slice of bread.

Serve with 1/2 cup rinsed and drained canned white beans tossed with 1 tablespoon chopped red onion, 1 teaspoon olive oil, and 1 tablespoon balsamic vinegar.

Lunch 3: Fiesta Salad

Hold the margarita and enjoy this fun, Mexican-inspired, healthy pregnancy meal.

Nutrition Facts

Calories: 542.7

Protein: 27.4g

Carbohydrate: 66.9g

Dietary Fiber: 20.7g

Total Sugars: 7.892g

Total Fat: 21.4g

Saturated Fat: 5.26g

Cholesterol: 20mg

Total Omega-3 FA: 0.401g

Calcium: 360mg

Iron: 5.411mg

Sodium: 394.3mg

Vitamin D: 0mcg

Folate: 415.8mcg

Folic Acid: 0mcg

Procedure

Top 2 cups chopped romaine lettuce with 1 cup canned black beans (rinsed and drained), half of a medium baked (or microwaved) sweet potato (cubed, with skin), 1/3 cup diced tomato, and 1/4 cup frozen and thawed corn kernels.

Drizzle with lime vinaigrette: 1 tablespoon lime juice, 1 tablespoon olive oil, 1/4 teaspoon chopped garlic, and salt and pepper to taste. Sprinkle with 1/4 cup of reduced-fat shredded Mexican blend cheese.

Lunch 4: Loaded Pesto Veggie Burger

Skip the fast food restaurant and make this burger at home to save time, money, and calories.

Nutrition Facts

Calories: 549.1

Protein: 33.2g

Carbohydrate: 55.4g

Dietary Fiber: 11.8g

Total Sugars: 13.3g

Total Fat: 22.2g

Saturated Fat: 7.257g

Cholesterol: 30.1mg

Total Omega-3 FA: 0.356g

Calcium: 413.5mg

Iron: 3.905mg

Sodium: 867.8mg

Vitamin D: 0.312 mcg

Folate: 125.3mcg

Folic Acid: 0mcg

Procedure

Cook a veggie burger according to the instructions. Using a grill pan sprayed with cooking spray, grill a thick slice of yellow onion and a Portobello mushroom cap.

Place veggie burger onto half of a whole wheat hamburger bun spread with 2 teaspoons of prepared pesto.

Top with a slice of Swiss cheese, Portobello mushroom, onion, and the second half of the bun. Serve with two carrots, cut into sticks, and dipped into 2 tablespoons of hummus.

Lunch 5: Panera Bread's "You Pick Two" Menu

Choosing a healthy pregnancy lunch when you're out can be daunting, but Panera Bread's "You Pick 2" menu makes it easy to eat right. Order half a Napa Almond Chicken sandwich, half a Strawberry Poppyseed & Chicken salad, and eat half an apple side.

Nutrition Facts

Calories: 550

Total Fat: 20g

Saturated Fat: 3g

Cholesterol: 60mg

Sodium: 780mg

Carbohydrate: 72.5g

Fiber: 7g

Protein: 29g

DINNER

Dinner 1: Stuffed Acorn Squash

Stuffed acorn squash has tons of nutrients that you need during pregnancy, but it's especially great for vegetarians.

Nutrition Facts

Calories: 641.7

Protein: 23.6g

Carbohydrate: 110.2g

Dietary Fiber: 16.2g

Total Sugars: 6.101g

Total Fat: 16.5g

Saturated Fat: 3.59g

Cholesterol: 6.8mg

Total Omega-3 FA: 438 g

Calcium: 362.5mg

Iron: 7.457mg

Sodium: 763.8mg

Vitamin C: 55.4mg

Folate: 198.2mcg

Folic Acid: 0 mg

Procedure

Cut one medium acorn squash in half horizontally; remove seeds. Place on a baking sheet sprayed with cooking spray, cut side down. Bake at 375 F for 45 minutes or until tender.

While squash is cooking, sauté 1/2 cup chopped onion, 1/2 cup chopped mushroom, 1/3 cup white beans, and one clove of chopped garlic in 2 teaspoons olive oil until soft, about 3–5 minutes.

Add 1 cup cooked wild or brown rice and 1 tablespoon chopped pistachios to the mixture and continue to stir until heated through, about 1 minute more. Set aside.

Remove the squash from the oven, stuff each half with the rice and bean mixture, then top each half with 2 tablespoons of

Parmesan cheese. Place in the
oven again and cook for an
additional 10 minutes.

Dinner 2: Parmesan Chicken Tenders with Marinara Dipping Sauce

When you're pregnant, doctors recommend at least 60 grams of protein each day, which shouldn't be a problem with a meal like this—it's packed with more than 50 grams!

Nutrition Facts

Calories: 649.2

Protein: 50.9g

Carbohydrate: 69.6g

Dietary Fiber: 10.7g

Total Sugars: 19.7g

Total Fat: 22.8g

Saturated Fat: 4.002g

Cholesterol: 92.5mg

Total Omega-3 FA: 0.222g

Calcium: 231.4mg

Iron: 3.678mg

Sodium: 1171mg

Vitamin C: 68.1mg

Folate: 86.5mcg

Folic Acid: 11.1 mcg

Procedure

To make this pregnancy recipe, preheat the oven to 475 F. Bread 5 ounces of chicken tenders by dipping in an egg wash made with two egg whites lightly beaten with a fork, then in 2 tablespoons of bread crumbs (preferably whole wheat) mixed with 1 tablespoon parmesan cheese, 1/2 teaspoon oregano, 1/4 teaspoon dry mustard, and 1/4 teaspoon garlic powder.

Bake chicken tenders on a wire rack or baking sheet sprayed with cooking spray for 15 minutes or until the chicken is cooked to 165 F internally. Serve with 4.5 ounces of baked Alexia sweet potato fries (about 18 fries) and 1 cup steamed broccoli drizzled with 1 teaspoon olive oil and a squeeze of lemon juice.

Dinner 3: Pork and Pineapple Kebobs

Throw some of these kebobs on the grill for a healthier alternative to standard BBQ fare.

Nutrition Facts

Calories: 640.6

Protein: 35.6g

Carbohydrate: 86.8g

Dietary Fiber: 15.2g

Total Sugars: 28.6g

Total Fat: 19.2g

Saturated Fat: 3.429g

Cholesterol: 71.4mg

Total Omega-3 FA: 0.187g

Calcium: 75.1mg

Iron: 4.212mg

Sodium: 366.8mg

Vitamin C: 103.2mg

Folate: 101.5mcg

Folic Acid: 0mcg

Procedure

First, cut 4 ounces of pork tenderloin or boneless top loin roast into 1.5-inch pieces. In a plastic baggie, add the juice of half a lime, a half clove of chopped garlic, 1/4 cup juice from pineapple canned in its juices, and 1 teaspoon olive oil. Let it marinate for about 30 minutes.

Next, cut half of the medium red bell pepper and one-fourth of a medium onion into 1-inch pieces. Thread pork, pepper, onion, and 1/2 cup canned pineapple chunks onto two skewers. Grill on a medium-high flame until pork is cooked to an internal temperature of 145 F.

Serve over 1.5 cups of cooked bulgur wheat tossed with 2 teaspoons olive oil, 1/8 teaspoon salt, and pepper to taste.

Dinner 4: Pizza and Salad

You've probably heard that you need more iron during pregnancy, but did you know that pizza can be a great place to find it?

Nutrition Facts

Calories: 640.4

Protein: 21.1g

Carbohydrate: 85.1g

Dietary Fiber: 13.6g

Total Sugars: 9.939g

Total Fat: 24.1g

Saturated Fat: 5.74g

Cholesterol: 15mg

Total Omega-3 FA: 0.087g

Calcium: 316mg

Iron: 8.733mg

Sodium: 1059mg

Vitamin C: 31.9mg

Folate: 92.3mcg

Folic Acid: 0mcg

Procedure

Heat an Amy's Organic Single Serve Pesto Pizza according to instructions.

Serve with a salad made with 1 cup mixed greens, half of sliced cucumber, 1 cup halved grape tomatoes, 1/2 cup canned chickpeas (rinsed and drained), 2 teaspoons olive oil, 2 teaspoons red wine vinegar, and garlic powder to taste.

Dinner 5: Healthier Nachos

Reduced-fat cheese and nonfat yogurt turn these nachos into a calcium-rich dinner for pregnancy.

Nutrition Facts

Calories: 656.8

Protein: 36.9g

Carbohydrate: 70.4g

Dietary Fiber: 11.9g

Total Sugars: 9.806g

Total Fat: 29g

Saturated Fat: 7.082g

Cholesterol: 30mg

Total Omega-3 FA: 0.44g

Calcium: 712.1mg

Iron: 4.461mg

Sodium: 1517mg

Vitamin C: 9.557mg

Folate: 140.6mcg

Folic Acid: 0mcg

Procedure

Layer 1-ounce corn chips with 1/3 cup kidney beans, 2 tablespoons chopped olives, and 1/4 cup shredded reduced-fat cheese.

Bake in the oven or toaster oven for about 10 minutes, or until all ingredients are hot and the cheese is melted.

Top with 1/2 cup shredded lettuce, 1/4 cup chopped tomatoes, 1/3 cup salsa, and 1/2 cup nonfat Greek yogurt.

CALCIUM-RICH SNACK
Calcium-Rich Snack 1: Crackers and Cheese

Soft cheeses may be off the menu while pregnant, but pasteurized and harder cheeses are a great way to get the extra calcium you need.

Nutrition Facts

Calories: 202.2

Protein: 7.205g

Carbohydrate: 24.8g

Dietary Fiber: 3.017g

Total Sugars: 4.561g

Total Fat: 8.394g

Saturated Fat: 0.855g

Cholesterol: 20mg

Total Omega-3 FA: 0.096g

Calcium: 133.2mg

Iron: 0.806mg

Sodium: 685mg

Vitamin C: 0.014mg

Folate: 7mcg

Folic Acid: 0mcg

Procedure

Spread five Triscuit Original Whole Grain Wheat Crackers with two Laughing Cow light cheese wedges and top with 1 tablespoon of dried cranberries.

Calcium-Rich Snack 2: Peachy Crunchy Yogurt

If you weren't a yogurt fan before pregnancy, now is an ideal time to convert. A nonfat yogurt will provide lots of protein and calcium but not a lot of sugar—a perfect combination for a pregnancy meal plan.

Nutrition Facts

Calories: 198.7

Protein: 15.7g

Carbohydrate: 25.2g

Dietary Fiber: 2.002g

Total Sugars: 19.1g

Total Fat: 3.854g

Saturated Fat: 0.503g

Cholesterol: 0mg

Total Omega-3 FA: 1.065g

Calcium: 216.2mg

Iron: 0.543mg

Sodium: 67.1mg

Vitamin C: 1.298mg

Folate: 9.679mcg

Folic Acid: 0mcg

Procedure

Grab a 6-ounce container of Chobani non-fat peach yogurt and mix with 2 teaspoons flaxseeds and 1 tablespoon granola.

Calcium-Rich Snack 3: Blueberry Almond Smoothie

Store-made smoothies can be loaded with sugar and are often lacking in nutrients.

Nutrition Facts

Calories: 202.5

Protein: 6.878g

Carbohydrate: 25.6g

Dietary Fiber: 5.758g

Total Sugars: 6.495g

Total Fat: 9.478g

Saturated Fat: 1.004g

Cholesterol: 0mg

Total Omega-3 FA: 0.045g

Calcium: 271.2mg

Iron: 1.835mg

Sodium: 68.4mg

Vitamin C: 1.895mg

Folate: 25.3mcg

Folic Acid: 0mcg

Procedure

Replace the traditionally high-in-sugar frozen yogurt—a smoothie staple—with unsweetened soy milk. Blend 3/4 cup frozen blueberries, 2 teaspoons almond butter, 1 teaspoon honey, and 3/4 cup unsweetened soy milk.

Calcium-Rich Snack 4: Smores Luna Bar

You can keep nutritional bars in your bag or car for a perfect on-the-go pregnancy snack. There are many bars on the market, but Luna Bars are made specifically for women with natural ingredients.

Nutrition Facts

Calories: 190

Protein: 8g

Carbohydrate: 28g

Fiber: 3g

Total Fat: 6g

Saturated Fat: 2.5g

Calcium: 78mg

Sodium: 115mg

Calcium-Rich Snack 5: Parmesan and Black Pepper Popcorn

The next time you want to munch on something salty in front of the TV, pick popcorn instead of potato chips. You'll satisfy your craving for some salt without the unhealthy fats found in greasy chips.

Nutrition Facts

Calories: 208.4

Protein: 8.357g

Carbohydrate: 30.5g

Dietary Fiber: 6.026g

Total Sugars: 0.091g

Total Fat: 5.114g

Saturated Fat: 1.731g

Cholesterol: 8.8mg

Total Omega-3 FA: 0.019g

Calcium: 111.3mg

Iron: 1.199mg

Sodium: 527.9mg

Vitamin C: 0.021mg

Folate: 1.01mcg

Folic Acid: 0mcg

Procedure

Toss 1/2 bag of 94% fat-free microwave popcorn with 2 tablespoons of parmesan cheese and black pepper to taste.

It's the perfect addition to a pregnancy meal plan!

SNACK

Snack 1: Peanut Butter Crackers

If you're not a big meat eater, finding other ways to get your protein is important, and peanut butter is full of it.

Nutrition Facts

Calories: 206.1

Protein: 7.748g

Carbohydrate: 20.9g

Dietary Fiber: 3.76g

Total Sugars: 5.208g

Total Fat: 11.3g

Saturated Fat: 1.647g

Cholesterol: 0mg

Total Omega-3 FA: 0.012g

Calcium: 44.2mg

Iron: 1.307mg

Sodium: 152.1mg

Vitamin C: 0mg

Folate: 11.8mcg

Folic Acid: 0mcg

Procedure

Evenly distribute 1 tablespoon of peanut butter on top of seven Kashi snack crackers, then top each with another cracker to make seven sandwiches.

Snack 2: Cashew Trail Mix

Heart-healthy unsaturated fats, like those found in nuts, help your baby's brain develop while keeping you full.

Nutrition Facts

Calories: 212

Protein: 5.763g

Carbohydrate: 30.4g

Dietary Fiber: 4.869g

Total Sugars: 11g

Total Fat: 8.675g

Saturated Fat: 1.571g

Cholesterol: 0mg

Total Omega-3 FA: 0.028g

Calcium: 15.4mg

Iron: 2.36mg

Sodium: 90.8mg

Vitamin C: 0.14mg

Folate: 13.2mcg

Folic Acid: 0mcg

Procedure

Mix 2 tablespoons of cashew pieces with 1/2 cup of whole-grain cereal like Nature's Path Heritage Flakes and four chopped dried apricot halves.

Snack 3: Hummus

Many dips and dressings are loaded with unhealthy fats and not many nutrients. For a pregnancy meal plan, dip veggies or pretzels in homemade hummus instead.

Nutrition Facts

Calories: 210

Protein: 6g

Carbohydrate: 32g

Fiber: 3g

Fat: 7g

Saturated fat: 1g

Sugars: 2g

Calcium: 24mg

Sodium: 597mg

Procedure

In a food processor, puree one 15-ounce can of rinsed and drained chickpeas, 3 tablespoons lemon juice, 3 tablespoons sesame tahini, 3 tablespoons water, 1 tablespoon olive oil, one clove of finely minced garlic, and 1/2 teaspoon salt.

Serve 1/4 cup with 1 ounce of pretzels.

Snack 4: Heat and Eat

Getting ready for a baby takes a lot of time and energy, which means you might not always have the time—or desire—to cook. So instead, try Amy's Light and Lean Pasta & Veggies dish for a microwavable but healthy snack.

Nutrition Facts

Calories: 210

Protein: 10g

Carbohydrate: 33g

Fiber: 3g

Fat: 5g

Saturated fat: 1.5g

Calcium: 150mg

Sodium: 470mg

Snack 5: Soup and Bread

Nutrition Facts

Calories: 200.7

Protein: 7.689g

Carbohydrate: 33.7g

Dietary Fiber: 3.416g

Total Sugars: 2.67g

Total Fat: 4.44g

Saturated Fat: 1.277g

Cholesterol: 3.283mg

Total Omega-3 FA: 0.892g

Calcium: 126.4mg

Iron: 2.498mg

Sodium: 625.9mg

Vitamin C: 0.723mg

Folate: 76.5mcg

Folic Acid: 4.82 mcg

Procedure

The next time you need a break, have a snack that forces you to sit down and just relax. For example, try 1 cup of ready-to-eat minestrone soup with 1/2 whole wheat English muffin topped with 1/2 teaspoon whipped butter.

TREAT

Treat 1: Dark Chocolate

Take a break from prepping the nursery and reward your hard work with a square of dark chocolate (about 1 ounce).

Because this treat is packed with natural antioxidants, you can satisfy your sweet tooth and meet your nutritional needs all at once.

Nutrition Facts

Calories: 168

Protein: 2g

Carbohydrate: 13g

Fiber: 3g

Fat: 12g

Saturated fat: 7g

Sodium: 6mg

Treat 2: Frozen Yogurt Pops

Every pregnancy meal plan should include a creamy frozen treat. We like Yasso's Sea Salt Caramel Frozen Greek Yogurt Pops.

Nutrition Facts

Calories: 100

Protein: 5g

Carbohydrate: 18g

Fiber: 0g

Fat: 0.5g

Saturated fat: 0g

Sugars: 16g

Sodium: 105mg

Treat 3: Smartfood Popcorn

Save the microwave popcorn for movie night and grab a 1-ounce bag of Smartfood popcorn when you're in a rush.

Bonus: This white cheddar-flavored popcorn is tasty, so you won't even need salt or butter.

Nutrition Facts

Calories: 160

Protein: 4g

Carbohydrate: 13g

Dietary Fiber: 2g

Total Sugars: 2g

Total Fat: 10g

Saturated Fat: 2g

Cholesterol: 5mg

Total Omega-3 FA: 0g

Calcium: 60mg

Iron: 0.5mg

Sodium: 240mg

Vitamin C: 0mg

Folate: 0mcg

Folic Acid: 0mcg

Treat 4: Creamy Strawberry Mousse

This five-ingredient dessert tastes decadent and is made with protein-rich Greek yogurt.

Nutrition Facts

Calories: 132

Protein: 8g

Carbohydrate: 25g

Fiber: 2g

Fat: 0g

Saturated fat: 0g

Sugar: 20g

Calcium: 10mg

Sodium: 29mg

Procedure

The night before you want to serve it, place 1 1/2 cups of nonfat vanilla-flavored Greek yogurt in a strainer over a bowl in the refrigerator to drain.

The next day, place the strained yogurt in a large bowl. Add 1 tablespoon honey, 3 tablespoons orange juice, and 2 teaspoons vanilla. Stir well.

Puree 10 ounces of frozen strawberries in a blender until smooth. Fold the strawberries into the yogurt. Taste for sweetness, adding more honey if you'd like. Divide between four glasses or bowls. Keep extras in the fridge for two or three days.

Treat 5: Fresh-Baked Chocolate Chip Cookie

Are you craving a chocolate chip cookie? To keep cookies fresh and portions small, instead of whipping up a whole batch, break out the refrigerated dough and bake one or two cookies at a time.

We like Nestlé Toll House's Original Chocolate Chip Cookies for a pregnancy meal plan!

Nutrition Facts

Calories: 90

Protein: 1g

Carbohydrate: 11g

Fiber: 0g

Fat: 4g

Saturated fat: 2g

Sugars: 7g

Sodium: 85mg

CONCLUSION

Embracing a Nourishing Pregnancy Journey

As we conclude our journey through the pages of "Pregnancy Cookbook with Nutritional Information," we reach the heart of what this book is all about—*the power of nutrition in guiding you toward a vibrant, healthy, and joy-filled pregnancy*. It has been my privilege to be your companion on this extraordinary path, where every bite you take contributes to the well-being of both you and your growing baby.

Throughout this book, I have explored the essential elements of prenatal nutrition, the nutritional building blocks of a healthy pregnancy, the significance of prenatal vitamins and supplements, and the advantages of a thoughtfully crafted pregnancy meal plan. I have also shared with you over 30 nourishing recipes, each a testament to the fusion of taste and nutrition, showcasing that eating well during pregnancy can be a delectable journey.

Now, as I bid farewell, I want to leave you with some essential takeaways:

1. **Knowledge is Power**: The foundation of a healthy pregnancy is knowledge. Understanding the importance of specific nutrients, making informed food choices, and being aware of your unique nutritional needs empowers you to navigate this journey with confidence.

2. **Balance is Key**: A balanced diet that encompasses a variety of nutrient-rich foods is the cornerstone of prenatal nutrition. Strive to create meals that incorporate a wide range of nutrients to support both your health and the development of your baby.

3. **Seek Professional Guidance**: Your healthcare provider is your invaluable partner in this journey. Regular check-ins and open communication will help ensure you receive the personalized medical advice you need.

4. **Adapt to Your Needs**: Every pregnancy is unique. Whether you have dietary preferences, restrictions, or are experiencing specific medical conditions, it's crucial to adapt your nutritional plan to meet your individual requirements.

5. **Embrace the Journey**: Pregnancy is a miraculous time in your life. Savor it. Celebrate it. Cherish it. While proper nutrition is essential, don't forget to revel in the wonder of the life you're nurturing.

As you embark on this journey, may you find the wisdom and inspiration within the pages of this book to make informed choices that nourish your body, your mind, and your spirit. Your pregnancy is not only about health but also about celebrating the beauty of creation and the love you hold for your future family.

This book has been my heartfelt offering to support you during this remarkable phase of your life. May your pregnancy be filled with vitality, joy, and the promise of a bright and healthy future for you and your little one. **Congratulations** on your journey, and may it be as nourishing and beautiful as the love that brought you here.

I HAVE A REQUEST

Dear **Reader**,

I hope this message finds you well. I am writing to kindly request your feedback and review of my recently published book, **"Pregnancy Cookbook With Nutritional Information."** Your thoughts and opinions are incredibly important to me, and I would greatly appreciate your honest review.

Your review will not only provide valuable insights but also help other potential readers make informed decisions about whether to explore the book. As a fellow reader, your perspective is highly regarded.

Here's how you can help:

- *Read the Book*: If you haven't already had the chance to read "[Book Title]," I'd be happy to provide you with a complimentary copy in your preferred format (eBook or paperback).
- *Share Your Review*: After reading the book, please take a moment to share your thoughts by leaving a review on popular book retail platforms, such as Amazon, Goodreads, or any other platform where you prefer to review books.
- *Be Honest and Constructive*: Your honest opinion is what matters most. Whether you loved the book or had some critical feedback, I welcome your insights. Constructive criticism is just as valuable as praise.
- *Spread the Word*: If you found the book enjoyable and enlightening, consider sharing your review with your friends and family or on your social media platforms to help others discover it.

Your support in providing a review will not only be deeply appreciated, but will also be instrumental in spreading the message and impact of the book. Your input will guide future readers and play a vital role in its success.

Thank you for taking the time to consider my request. Your support means a great deal to me, and I am grateful for your willingness to share your thoughts on **"Pregnancy Cookbook With Nutritional Information."**

Wishing you an enriching reading experience, and I look forward to hearing from you.

Warm regards,

Kimberley Garcia

ADDITIONAL RESOURCES

Dear Reader, I am here again:

Thank you for your support and interest in "Pregnancy Cookbook With Nutritional Information". If you enjoyed this book and are looking for more valuable resources and engaging content, I would recommend some of my books that you might find intriguing:

1. "Best Parenting Book For Kids With ADHD": An ADHD Parenting Guide for Raising Hyperactive Kids, Dealing with Behavioral Issues, and Supporting Explosive Children
2. "Finding Relief": 10 Home Remedies To Relieve Menstrual Cramps
3. "Successful Parenting Of Kids With Autism": Easy Steps To Raising Brilliant Autistic Kids
4. "Single Mom's Pregnancy Guide": A Comprehensive Guide For Single Mothers

To explore these books, please visit my Author Central Page on Amazon. **You can scan the QR code below or click the link to visit my Author Central:**

https://www.amazon.com/author/kimberley_garcia

Your continued support means the world to me, and I am committed to providing you with valuable information and inspiration on your journey as a woman.

Thank you for being a part of this community, and I hope my books continue to bring you joy and empowerment.

Warm regards,
Kimberley Garcia

PS: Don't forget to check out my Author Central page on Amazon to discover more of my books. Your feedback and reviews are always appreciated!